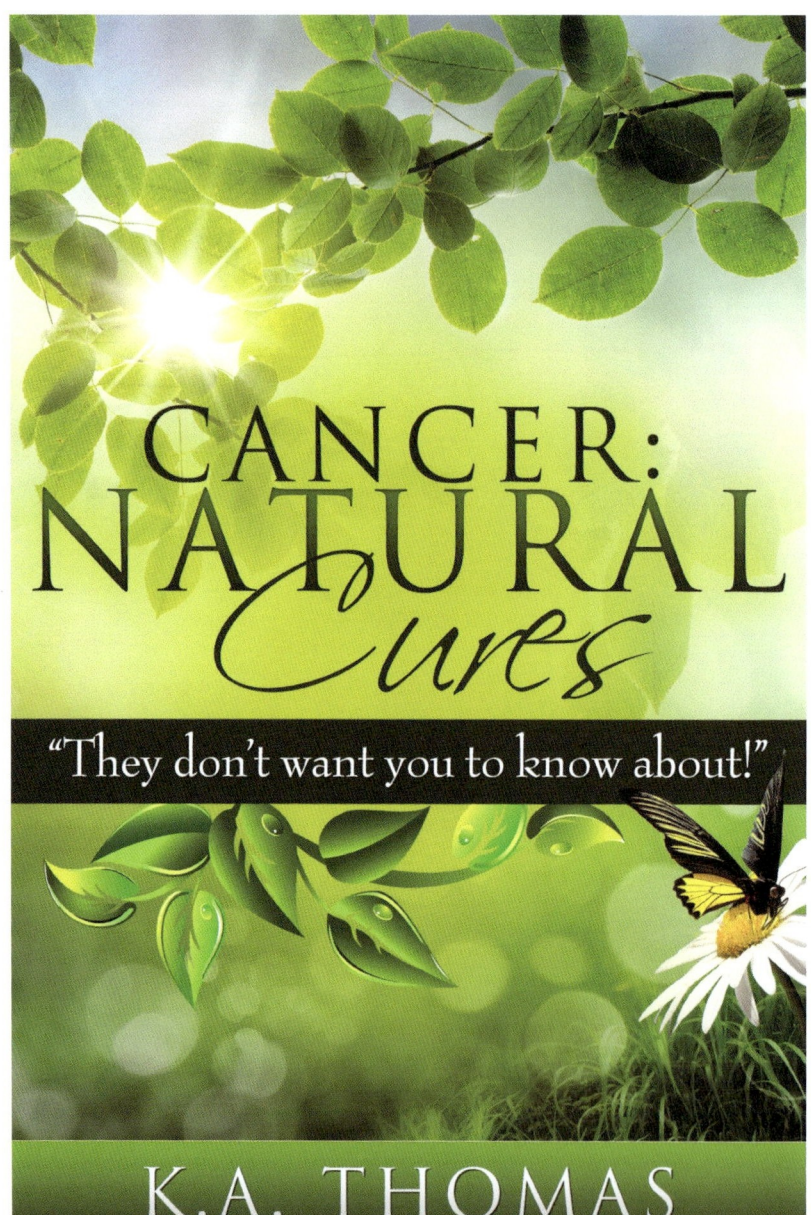

CANCER:

NATURAL CURES

"They don't want you to know about!"

All rights reserved. No part of this publication may be reproduced, distributed, or transmitted in any form or by any means, including photocopying, recording, or other electronic or mechanical methods, without the prior written permission of the publisher, except in the case of brief quotations embodied in critical reviews and certain other noncommercial uses permitted by copyright law.

Copyright © 2013 By K.A. Thomas

Table of Contents

Disclaimer 5
Dedication 6
R.I.P. John Joseph Fletcher – May 11, 1942 – May 31, 2013 6
Introduction 8
The Cancer Gene 10
Understanding Body pH 14
What Cancer Thrives On 18
4 Main Causes of Cancer (most illnesses) 21
Natural Cures 23
Baking Soda/Black Strap Molasses 25
The Gerson Therapy 31
The Budwig Protocol 34
Laetril – B17 – Apricot Seeds 39
Intravenous Vitamin C 42
The Power of Barley Leaves Extracts 45
The Power of Essential Oils 50
Immune Boosters 55
Diet, Nutrition & Detox 58
Essiac Tea 63
Testing 66
The Reality of Western Medicine 68
Other Protocols & Links 74
Conclusion 76

Disclaimer

Unfortunately I have to add a Disclaimer to this book as the FDA makes this mandatory.

This book is for educational purposes only. I am not a doctor.

This book has been written and published strictly for informational purposes, and in no way should be used as a substitute for advice from your own health care professionals.

Therefore, you must not consider educational material found here as a replacement for consultation with oncologists or any type of medical practitioners.

Dedication

I dedicate this book to my loving father John Joseph Fletcher, whom was my greatest teacher and motivator. He provided the most profound impact on my life, in everyway possible. As my promise to him, my journey is to educate people on natural alternative healing, opposed to only relying on traditional western medicine.

R.I.P. John Joseph Fletcher – May 11, 1942 – May 31, 2013

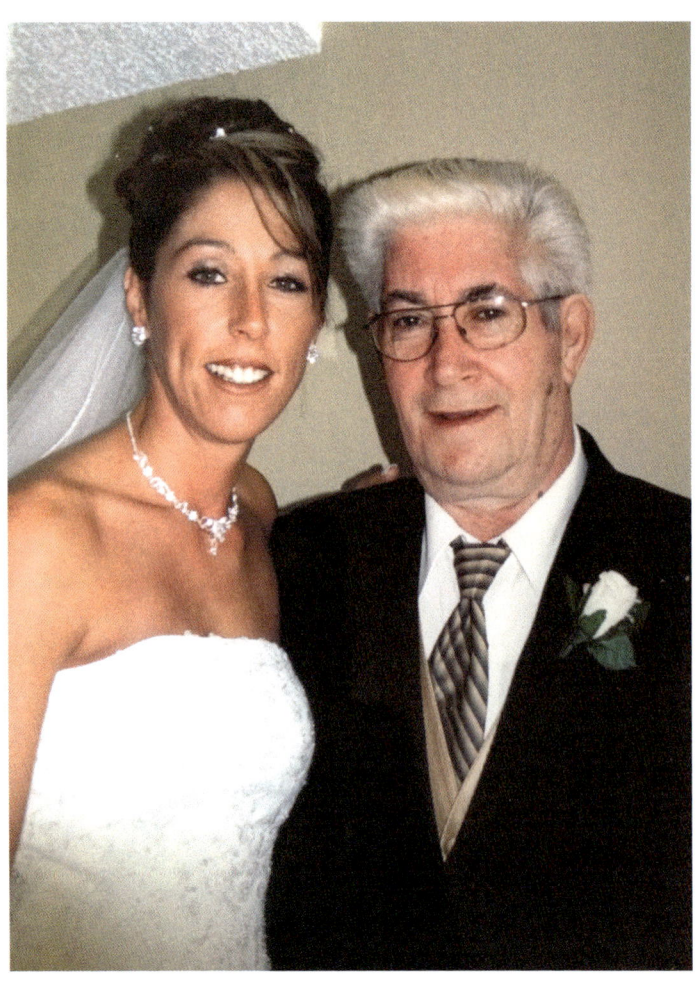

Introduction

After my father was diagnosed with late Stage 4 Lung Cancer I literally dropped both of my 2 jobs, moved both my parents in with my family and started taking care of him. It wasn't even a thought but just a quick action that kicks in. I became his fulltime caregiver and advocate. One of my two living rooms was literally turned into a hospital room as he became sicker throughout the months.

There were many fights with the doctors, the nurses, pharmacologists and oncologists as many mistakes were made due to simple oversights during the 8 month ordeal.

Due to being diagnosed very late the only option his oncologist gave him was 5 days of radiation treatment to reduce the pain. Over the last 10 months I have studied everything in regard to alternative medicine, natural cures, what causes disease, spoken to countless of cancer survivors that have cured themselves naturally rather than depending on western medicine and cried and smiled with many along the way.

When people are told, "You have cancer, you should start to get your affairs in order" they automatically switch on the death sentence within their brain and that is exactly what my father did.

In his mind he was given a death sentence, an expiry date and I personally would not stand for it. I became his cheerleader !

Watching the man I first fell in love with as a young child slowly die in front of me was heart wrenching. Feeding him, helping him to the washroom when he could no longer walk, changing his depends, administering subcutaneous injections for the pain when he couldn't swallow anymore and trying to calm him down when the delirium and hallucinations set in were some of the hardest things I had to endure, but somewhere you find the strength to do whatever you have to do.

He died exactly 8 months after diagnosis from Hypercalcemia which caused cardiac arrest (May 31, 2013) and I promised my father when he still had his mind that it would be my journey to educate the public on natural alternative healing. That cancer does not have to be a death sentence. It's your battle, it's how you plan on dealing with it, mind, body and spirit.

I realize that sometimes there is just no chance depending on the stage, complication and mindset, although everyone should be aware that there are options other than radiation, chemotherapy and western medicine that's offered so easily on a silver platter.

Today cancer seems to be like the flu. Everywhere you turn around someone has been diagnosed with cancer or some kind of malady which is quite frightening. Why is this happening? Have you really thought hard about this? What has changed in the last several decades for this to happen? I know. Do you ?

So why listen to me? I am just a mother, wife and daughter that truly cares about what is happening in today's society, to our loved ones. I am only one voice but I am making sure that people hear it and even if it only reaches a few that will make me happy. The things I have discovered have made me sick to death and having to deal with this first hand, do research for months on end, having not slept for several days at a time have made my drive that much more stronger to have my voice heard.

But last and most important, I am NOT a doctor which I believe is the most vital factor because you can trust my insight considering it's coming from someone that has gone through it first hand with a loved one and not handing out a prescription for a buck.

Some will disagree with what I write in this book and others will not and that is fine as everyone is entitled to their opinion and I respect that. I hope that you at least take away something that will help you in some way and please feel free to reach out and contact me if you wish on my facebook fanpage.

https://www.facebook.com/LivingNaturallyRaw

The Cancer Gene

Every one of us has cancer cells in our body, and having a strong immune system (natural killer cells) is normally successful in destroying them, so the key to fighting cancer is making sure you keep your immune system strong.

Disease or Cancer of any kind is a warning that your immune system has been weakened in one way or another and that your lifestyle and diet needs to be changed.

You cannot just treat the symptoms, you have to find the route cause and treat the cause in order to remain at an optimum health.

When my father was first diagnosed in October, I went crazy reading everything I could get my hands on. Medical journals, natural remedies, success stories, anything I could find. It was my time to put myself aside and focus 150% on my father and try and save his life.

I stumbled upon a blog of a man named Vernon Johnston. My graphic designer had sent me the link once he learned about my father's cancer. I read the blog intensively along with all the other success stories that followed his.

I was determine to speak to these people prior to putting my father on any protocol. I tracked down 3 Cancer survivors within the second month, Vernon, Colleen and Don and spoke to them each in great length by the ending of November.

One evening when speaking with Vernon, he had explained that a Molecular Physicist had contacted him and explained that he belonged to this 'Think Tank' of physicists and scientists where they discuss the alleged unknown.

The is the email that was written to Vernon by this "Ghost Scientist" and then Vernon emailed me a copy which follows below.

I just read your story, and watched the protocol video you made for youtube. I am a Molecular Physicist with a background in advanced molecular design and engineering. My mother was diagnosed with terminal cancer over 25 years ago. Her cancer stemmed from Sarcoidosis; my mother was one of the research patients at the Mayo Clinic in Rochester, MN who helped the Mayo pinpoint the disease and to classify it for the medical journals.

During the course of my young adult life, I strived to understand this tiny little gene that was affecting my mother, and why it seemed that the medical community could do nothing to reverse its devastating effects on her. As a research scientist I dove in with both feet and was looking to get at the core of the problem.

Here is what I found and what would save my mother's life and why she is still alive to this day and why you are still alive today.

Cancer gene & cell:

The cancer cell stems from a very short strand of DNA within the helix, its number is 274. This is a very interesting gene strand as every human being contains this specific strand of DNA. This particular gene strand is triggered by a lack of oxygen in the body. Once the body reaches a particular low oxygen environment this little gene wakes up and comes to life forming cancer cells. These cancer cells which are carried throughout the body by erythrocytes to varying places where they are then deposited and begin to take hold.

The sodium bi-carbonate solution you are taking is allowing the thinning of your erythrocyte wall therefore your erythrocytes is able to take in more oxygen and carry it throughout your body. When the oxygen atom comes into contact with a cancer cell it kills the cell and becomes dormant. The reason for explaining how and why the cancer cells are growing within your body is to explain to you why you are seeing an effect in change using sodium bi-carbonate as a supplement. When you are able to boost the oxygen level within your body the cancer cells begin to die off as they are not able to survive in an oxygen enriched environment.

Having figured out how to kill the cell I designed a protocol for my mother using purely organic compounds. These compounds are easy to get, easy to assemble and takes little or no time at all to see results. . . . . All I can tell you is my mother and many hundreds of other people I have helped to make this organic substance, are still alive and happy today. I do not sell anything, never have never will…I will also let you know that the medical community at large within cancer research know that this organic compound works to kill off all of the cells quickly and efficiently within the matter of a few days not weeks depending on the location of growth of the cell.

If you are interested in speaking with me about it I would love to have a conversation with you and explain to you how it works and why.

Respectfully. . .

Now after many conversations and research what you have to understand is simply one thing. Cancer cells can not survivor in an oxygenated body. Once your bodies oxygen lowers to a certain level that is when the cancer cell gene awakens and starts to invade the body and cancer starts to develop.

Let's take this a little further to help understand the process.

Dr. Warburg won his first Nobel Prize in 1931 for proving cancer is caused by a lack of oxygen respiration in cells. In newly formed cells, low levels of oxygen damage respiration enzymes so these cells cannot produce energy using oxygen. Ultimately these cells can turn cancerous.

Of course cancer has countless secondary causes, but it is factual that the primary cause is low cellular oxygenation levels.

Low or poor oxygenation comes from a buildup of carcinogens and many other toxins within and or around cells, which blocks and then damages the cellular oxygen respiration function.

The clumping of red blood cells slows down the bloodstream, and restricts the flow into the capillaries. Again this causes low or poor oxygenation.

The prime cause of cancer is the replacement of the respiration of oxygen in normal body cells by fermentation of sugar. All normal body cells meet their energy needs by respiration of oxygen, whereby cancer cells meet their energy needs most by fermentation.

To further understand, fermentation allows these cells to survive, but they can no longer perform any function in the body or communicate with the body in which it needs to in order to function properly. So these cells then can only multiply and grow.

A more accurate statement would be, they degrade into cancer cells that no longer server your body, but live to survive and destroy.

Part of Dr. Warburg's theory stated that cancer with the highest growth rates had the highest fermentation rates. The slower it grew, the less it used fermentation to produce energy.

Vernon beat cancer by restoring his bodies pH back to a normal state just by taking baking soda and molasses protocol and this has worked by many.

When you can keep your bodies pH at a normal balance you have won the game. It's seem's easy enough to do although it's alot harder than you think when you already have a diagnosis.

The next chapter will fully explain our bodies pH which is vitally essential to understand and live at the healthiest levels.

Understanding Body pH

To understand body pH and it's role with regulating your health, you must first understand "Alkaline vs. Acidic pH.

pH (potential of hydrogen) is a measure of the acidity or alkalinity of a solution. In the human body this is tested through the pH of urine and or salvia. However, it really reflects the pH of the blood. The pH of a solution is measured on a scale from 0 to 14. The higher pH indicated, the greater oxygen richness (alkaline). The lower pH indicates oxygen deprivation (acidic). When a solution is neither acid nor alkaline it has a pH of 7 which is considered neutral.

The ideal body pH is 7.35.

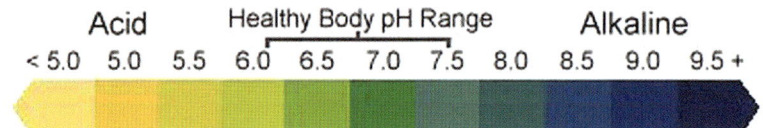

The Acid Alkaline imbalance within our bodies

One of the most common causes among people who have been stricken with disease comes down to pH imbalance.

When your body is over acidity this becomes extremely dangerous as it weakens all body immune systems, as apposed to a pH balanced body which allows the body to function normal and resist disease. When you look at a healthy body it is maintaining the adequate alkaline which it needs to meet your bodies emergency demands.

When we have excess acids that must be stabilized our alkaline reserves are eaten up leaving the body in a weakened state and vulnerable. The fact is, a pH balanced diet, according to many leading experts is the vital key to a long healthy lifestyle. Disease being caused by an acid alkaline imbalance is not new to the medical world, and now people are starting to take notice and are taking hold to understand how to maintain a healthy body pH on their own.

You can monitor your own body pH levels in the comfort of your home with pH strips which you can purchase just about anywhere.

The majority of people that have an unbalanced pH are acidic. When your body pH is acidic it forces the body to borrow minerals which include sodium, calcium, potassium and magnesium from our vital organs and bones to neutralize the acid and to safely remove it from the body. Due to this stress being caused, the body can suffer severe and prolonged damage due to high acidity.

Low pH (acidic) affects your health at the cellular level and can cause problems such as:

Poor sleep

Poor digestion

Premature aging

Acceleration of free radical damage, contributing to cancerous mutations

Osteoporosis

Low energy and chronic fatigue

Bladder and kidney conditions

Weight gain, diabetes and obesity just to name few

Restoring the body's pH

It's important to understand that when your body pH is acidic it is extremely difficult to absorb minerals and nutrients properly, but not impossible.

Step 1

Start paying attention to the foods you eat so you can understand your eating habits. Start consuming more alkaline-forming foods. Your daily ratio should be the 80/20 rule; 80% alkaline foods to 20% acid-forming foods. This will be the best tactic to start re-balancing an acidic body pH.

Some acid-forming foods include dairy products, meat, cooked foods, sugars, refined flour and salts. Some great Alkaline-forming foods that you can include in your diet today are fruits and vegetables such as onions, beets, broccoli, lemons, carrots, leeks, mangoes, asapargus, melons, sweet potatoes, almonds and flax seeds just to name a few.

NOTE : If you have been diagnosed with cancer, stay away from all acid forming foods as much as you possibly can.

Step 2

Drink lemon water everyday, several times a day. I have included this in my daily ritual as it tastes great and is very high in alkaline. Lemons, grapefruit and limes are high alkaline-forming foods. The great thing about lemon water is it will enhance liver function and it provides the important antioxidant vitamin C which fights free radicals which damage healthy cells.

Step 3

Chlorophyll significantly raises the pH of foods so that they are more alkaline forming. Foods that are rich in chlorophyll (which give the plants their green color) are asparagus, cucumbers, green beans, bell peppers, peas, sprouts, parsley and all leafy greens.

Step 4

Everyone has some stressors that they deal with on a daily basis. Managing your stress can also encourage alkalinity and promotes a positive attitude. Take time for yourself to do the things you enjoy, even if it's only for 15 minutes. Some examples may include yoga, meditation, a light walk and deep breathing exercises.

The truth is everyone has different nutrient requirements, but we all share one thing in common – we need to have alkaline blood to stay healthy!

You have to understand that at the end of the day, YOU are in control of your health and you can start making decisions to start living healthier today.

As the saying goes, "You Are What You Eat"!

What Cancer Thrives On

I will be short and to the point on this chapter as it boils my blood and I would ramble which you don't want.

Just to explain, the reason why this subject makes me so angry is that our health system, hospitals and dieticians are constantly feeding our loved ones that have been afflicted with this awful disease, these acidic foods knowing that they specifically speed up the growth of cancer cells.

Here are some of main foods that feed cancer cells and speed up growth.

Sugar is the number one food item that feeds cancer and allows the cells to grow and divide at a rapid rate. Highly processed carbohydrates are sugars. By eliminating sugar and refined carbohydrates from the diet this cuts off the food supply to the cancer cells. Sugar substitutes, refined flour and trans-fatty acids damage the body and numerous studies link them to cancer.

Also be aware that refined carbohydrates are turned rapidly into sugar in the stomach to produce what body builders and others refer to as a "sugar rush".

Dairy and all mucus-forming foods should also be avoided. Cancer feeds on mucus, especially in the colon. Eliminating milk and milk based products helps starve cancer cells.

Processed foods, carbonated beverages, coffee, alcohol, chlorine and fluoride fall into the category of foods and substances that interfere with healing and fuel the cancer's growth.

Remember that an acid environment fuels cancer growth. Meat based diets make the body acidic. You must understand that meat protein is difficult to digest and requires a lot of energy and digestive enzymes. Undigested meat becomes putrefied and leads to toxic buildup.

Cancer cells contain a hard protein wall which needs to be broken down. By cutting out meat this frees more enzymes to attack the protein walls of the cancer cells and allows the bodies natural killer cells to destroy them.

Stress is a known factor to put the body in a acidic state.

I can't stress enough that cancer cells thrive in an acidic environment. Get your body back to a natural pH balance !

Just to give you a simple example the medical world is well aware that cancer feeds off sugar. The great old "PET SCAN" which they insert the dye containing sugar to see where the cancer is active. Why are they injecting a sugar based dye to see where the cancer cells are active? Because they know CANCER FEEDS OFF SUGAR! So why do they continue to feed it to us in the hospital ?

Your diet should consist of an alkaline diet meaning 80% of fresh vegetables and juice, whole grain seeds, little fruits, seeds and nuts.

Physicians and oncologists state that cancerous cells feed on sugar. They understand that cancer thrives in an acidic environment but they continue to feed their patients table sugar, the red meats, dairy products, coffee, candy, soda pop, white flour products that the hospitals are providing their cancer patients every single day.

Either it's just too costly to provide the cancer patient with an alkaline diet (nutritious) meal or they are just part of this greedy thing we call the all mighty dollar or just plain out lazy.

When my father and I met with the nutritionist, the meal plan she presented us was mind blowing. My jaw literally dropped on the floor. Why aren't these so called industry experts being trained properly?

The reality is, Cancer is big, big money. In fact a 300 billion dollar industry and if something so simple as baking soda and some of the other natural cures we will discuss were to have the word "Cure" on it, oh my god the Big Pharma Companies would fold literally overnight.

4 Main Causes of Cancer (most illnesses)

Cause Number 1 – A Weak Immune System

Usually caused by a severe negative emotional shock (death in the family, divorce, family problems, financial setbacks, etc.) overworked and run down over an extended period of time, pessimistic negative thinking most of the time, lack of rest, and improper nutrition that reinforces the immune system. Ed Sopcak a cancer researcher in United States consulted with over 30,000 cancer patients. He concluded "most all the cancer patients I have spoken with had a major stress in their life six months to 3 years before they were diagnosed with cancer.

Cause Number 2 – Toxins

Such as dangerous chemicals (in the workplace, home or garden), microbes, parasites and fungus, etc. The late Dr. Hulda Clark who examined and treated thousands of cancer patients stated that "all cancer patients have both isopropyl alcohol (as found in many body care and household cleaning products) and the intestinal fluke (parasites, worms) in their liver".

Cause No 3 - Improper Diet

Cancer thrives in an "acidic" environment (low pH). A regular consumption of "acidic foods" such as soda pops, chips (crisps), coffee, store bought pastries, processed foods, deep fried foods (French fries, donuts), prepared meats (hot dogs, sausages, bacon, ham) fast foods, food additives, aspartame etc. contribute to cancer.

Cause No 4 - Oxygen Deprivation

Tran's fats (margarine, refined vegetable oils) used in deep fried foods and processed foods (mayonnaise, refined vegetable oils) actually suffocate the cells when ingested depriving the body of life giving oxygen. You should only be using "cold pressed" natural oils, such as flaxseed oil, coconut oil, etc.

It may be a combination of all four of these "causes" or one in particular that a cancer patient can pinpoint as their main reason for having cancer. One thing for sure, your diet, lifestyle and state of mind are absolutely critical to prevent and/or win this battle. And another thing for sure is you need to "remove" these four causes to win the battle against cancer.

Natural Cures

Natural cures are everywhere around us. For some reason we have decided to ignore them or just not eductate ourselves about them and rely on our "Practising Physicians" recommendations due to our faith and trust in them. The reason I state "practicing" is that is how I feel. We are the ginny pigs that they are practicing on.

"Here's your prescription. Next!"

For one they never try and investigate the underlying cause of why or where the disease has stemmed from and most do not have a clue about basic nutrition. They are too busy rushing you into surgery or to start radiation or chemotherapy. When was the last time your doctor or oncologist asked you about your diet and lifestyle ?

After I started my research when my father was first diagnosed, a large world opened up in front of me that I have never paid much attention to. I was shocked and stunned at the information that I had found, actually I was extremely "pissed off" to put it lightly.

I think there is now over 350 cures dated as I write this book and all if not most have been deemed by the medical world as quackery or their studies diluted the protocol so it shows in their data and clinic journals proven not to work.

How and why would the medical world state that they have not found a cure yet when there have been so many sitting in front us for years, and most for only a fraction of the cost. The reason is simple, there is no money in cures that cost under 100$ and there are no repeat visits or prescriptions.

There are very few doctors that will come forward and truly speak out loud announcing that there is a cure and when this happens they are ostracized by the medical world as a quack, go to jail or have their medical license taken away.

No wonder there are so many doctors that keep quiet and will not share what they know.

In late October my graphic designer sent me a link to a cancer protocol to check out, so I went digging. I think I read the blog about 5 times that night just so it would fully sink in.

Vernon Johnston was diagnosed with class IV Aggressive Prostate Cancer that had spread to the bones. He decided to treat himself with a protocol called the "Baking Soda / Black Strap Molasses.

He is now cancer free and has been for many years. Before I started my father on any protocol I needed to speak to several survivors to have some hope, so I tracked down three people including Vernon that used the protocol with success.

I spoke to Vernon on several occasions, along with Colleen whom had breast cancer and Don Porter whom also had late stage prostate cancer. All are alive and well today thanks to sodium bicarbonate. I actually still text Colleen regularly and just recently spoke to Vernon again just prior to my father's passing.

Baking Soda/Black Strap Molasses

First off the pH of baking soda in pure water is 8.2. This protocol is an extremely effective way to raise your body pH quickly.

Here is a quick understanding of how the two (bs/molasses) work together;

Cancer cells eat up the sugar so when you encourage the intake of sugar it's like sending in a Trojan horse. The sugar of the molasses is not going to encourage the growth of the cancer colonies because the baking soda is going to kill the cells before they have a chance to grow.

The molasses targets the cancer cells (which consume 15 times more glucose than normal cells) and the baking soda, which is dragged into the cancer cell by way of the molasses, being very alkaline forces a rapid shift in pH killing the cells.

Cancer cells become dormant at a body pH of 7.0 - 7.5 and kills cancer cells at 8.0 to 8.5.

Day 1

1 Teaspoon of BS (baking soda) with 2 teaspoons of BSM (black strap molasses) mixed with 1 cup of water, twice daily. Heat in pot at low temperature for 5 minutes and stir until fully combined to create your "Trojan Horse".

Day 2

Repeat Day 1
Include Deep Breathing Exercises
30 Deep breathing exercises 10 x per day or more if you can (oxygen kills cancer cells)

Day 3

Repeat Day 1 and deep breathing exercises

Day 4

Repeat Day 1 and deep breathing exercises
Your goal is to get your body pH to 8.0 - 8.5 and hold it there for 4 to 5 days

Day 5

2 teaspoons of BS with 2 teaspoons of BSM with 1 cup of water twice per day.

You may experience some mild nausea which is a good sign. This is a signal that the dead cancer cells are being discarded by your body.
Continue with the deep breathing exercises

Day 6

Repeat Day 5 with your deep breathing exercises

Day 7

Repeat Day 5 with your deep breathing exercises

Day 8

Double dose 3 x a day to up you pH level if you can tolerate it. Your body will tell you. Start taking 200 mg of Potassium supplements which is extremely important!)
Continue with your deep breathing exercises

Day 9

Repeat Day 8 with breathing exercises and 200 to 300mg of potassium supplements

Day 10

Cut back to 2 x a day (day 5 procedure); continue with breathing exercises and potassium supplements

Day 11

Cut back to 1.5 teaspoons of BS with 1 teaspoon of BSM and 1 cup of water. Continue with deep breathing and potassium supplements.

Break for 7 to 14 days and repeat again if necessary

Some of the added supplements are added below to go with this protocol:

Coral Calcium - 3000mg
Vitamin D# 10,000 IU's
Spirulina and Chlorella (super foods)
Milk Thistle - 1000 mg (immune booster)
Organic and juicing diet to rebuild the immune system
Co Q10 200mg
Potassium 200mg
pH strips to monitor your ph levels

You should always take the protocol (BS / BSM) 2 hours before or after eating.

You should take your pH test once in the morning when first waking both urine and saliva

Track everything for the entire 11 days

Now Vernon, Colleen and Don have all used this protocol which saved their lives. I did have my father on this protocol just the one time although he had so many other complications that required hospitalization which halted everything in its track. I am in the process of writing my memoir of our 8 month journey which will explain what he and I went through in great detail.

More Baking Soda / Blackstap Molasses proof :

COUNTY DOCTOR CURES CANCER WITH BAKING SODA & MAPLE SYRUP

ASHVILLE, N.C. – "There's not a tumor on God's green Earth that can't be licked with a little baking soda and maple syrup!" That's the astonishing claim of controversial folk healer Jim Kemun—who says his simple home remedy can stop and reverse the growth of deadly cancers.

The 75-year-old former truck driver has no medical degree and authorities are demanding that he stop dispensing his "wonder drug" –or face a prison sentence.

But his loyal patients swear by the man they fondly call "Dr. Jim"—and say he's a miracle worker.

"Dr. Jim cured me of lung cancer," declares farmer Ian Rodhouse, 64. "Those other doctors told me I was a goner and had less than six months to live.

"But the doc put me on his mixture—and in a couple of months, the caner was gone. It didn't even show up on X-rays!"

The gentle, silver-haired grandfather—who has been preparing home remedies since 1954—says he first hit upon the miracle cure in the mid-1970's, when he was treating a family plagued by breast cancer.
"There were five sisters in the family and all of them passed away from the big C by age 50—except one," he recalls.

"I asked if there was anything different in her diet. She told me she was partial to sipping maple syrup and baking soda.

"I figured, let me try it out on some of my other patients."

Since then, "Dr. Jim" has dispensed his mixture to more than 200 patients diagnosed with terminal cancer. Amazingly, he claims that of that number, 185 lived at least 15 more years—and nearly half enjoyed a complete remission of their disease.

"You tell me about another treatment that works that good!" he demands proudly.

Medical experts are less enthusiastic. "This man is a quack, plain and simple," blasts an official at a state medical association. "We intend to see that he is arrested for practicing medicine without a license."

Until that happens, Dr. Jim vows to keep prescribing his treatment: "I'm just going to keep on saving lives."

Here is a picture of the original news article below :

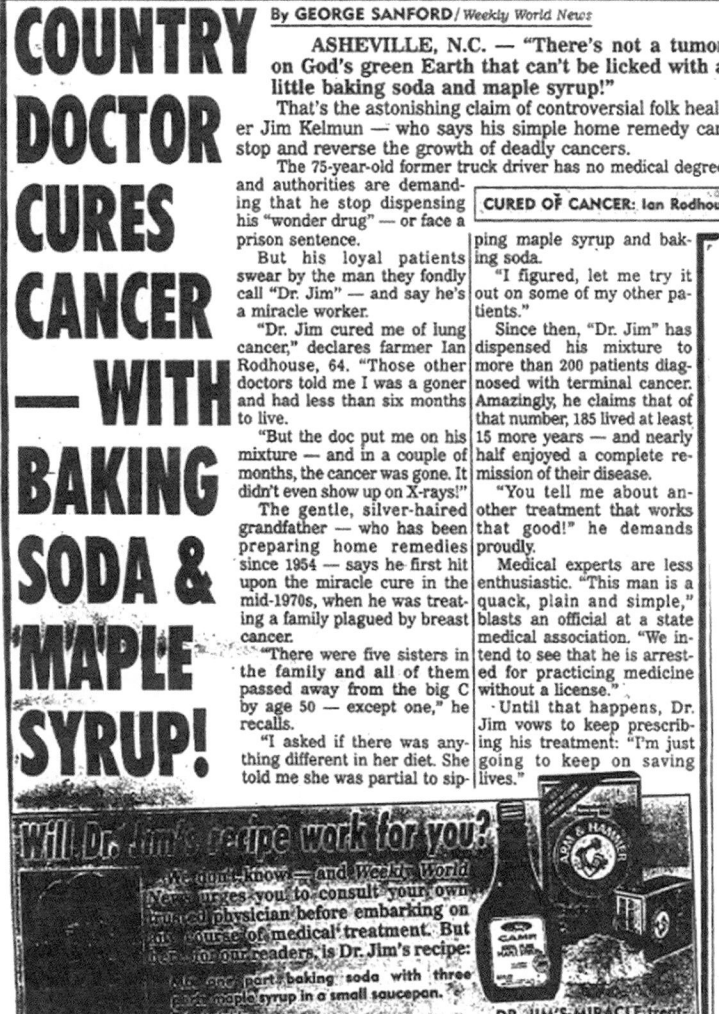

This protocol has WORKED for many! Do your research, it's out there.

The Gerson Therapy

The Gerson Instution was founded by Dr. Gerson's daughter, Charlotte Gerson in 1977. They are located in San Diego, California and are dedicated to educating and training alternative, non-toxic treatment for cancer and all other chronic degenerative diseases.

Charlotte's father, Max Gerson developed the natural treatment in the late 1920's. Their methods allow the body to activate it's ability to heal itself by way of organic, vegetarian diet, raw juices, coffee enemas and natural supplements.

The Gerson Therapy treats the underlying causes of disease which are mostly toxicity and nutritrional deficiency. They treat the body as a whole, rather than the specific condition or symptom.

They have been renouned for recovering so called incurable diseases. I recommend that you research their site and become educated and learn more on your own.

They offer several options of which you can be treated in one of their clinics or you can have the option of treating yourself in the comfort of your home.

They have hundreds of testimonials of cancer survivors and are highly recommended by many.

Here is one below :

Kent Gardner at the age of forty six was diagnosed with both cancer of the esophagus and larynx. He was given an 8% chance of a five year survival rate from his oncologist.

This is what Kent stated in the Gerson Therapy Newsletter:

"I bought the Gerson Therapy book (A Cancer Therapy: Results of Fifty Cases), read it two times in less than twenty days, then decided, what do I have to lose? I knew I was dying. The coffee

enemas were a mental hurdle I had to overcome, but once I experienced one of them, I could feel a difference in the boosting of my health and realized their importance," Kent Gardner wrote for the Gerson Healing Newsletter.

"After about one and a half months, the swelling was way down, and the tumor was dead," he continues. "Reducing in size weekly, it was rotting in my throat. Frankly, it felt like hell! This thing now rotting produced a constant, horrible smell unlike anything I had ever experienced- even after working for twenty-four years a taxidermist!

"Still doing the Gerson Therapy faithfully, about two and a half months later, as I was locking my car to walk into a local hardware store, the dead tumor fluttered for about two seconds, then as I swallowed I felt it break free. I sort of staggered into the store, feeling panicked. I broke into a profuse sweating and starting losing consciousness. I fell to my knees in a series of convulsions, and I knew I was in trouble," Mr. Gardner asserts.

"Thinking about this situation later, I realized the tumor had fallen into my stomach, where it mixed with digestive juices, producing ammonia poisons and gases. I should have tried to throw it up, but ego, and not being able to think clearly, didn't allow me to vomit publicly. To this day, "admits Mr. Gardner, "I don't remember or know how I managed to make it back to my car and then drive home, which was a twenty-minute ride. For the next five days I was totally bedridden.

"I took three coffee enemas a day; my wife helped me, doing all that was necessary. The tumor's toxic effects were manifold- headaches, vomiting, bad abdominal cramps, and many other troubles," the taxidermist states. "I was in an awful state of absolute illness!

"But on the sixth day I felt better and was able to walk around. I have been walking on water ever since. Because of that experience, I have done my homework and am experientially educated far beyond my I.Q., concerning the human body and nutrition," Kent Gardner says. "All living cells and organisms on this planet need water, food and air. It is the quality, not the quantity that determines perfect health, or disease. You can't trash and pollute your body and expect to have perfect health. What all of us need are daily coffee enemas, something I do on a regular basis - cancer or not."

The Gerson Therapy is highly recommended by many and has helped saved thousand of lives. They truly care about the underlying cause and then treating it from the inside out.

Charlotte Gerson is an absolute rockstar when it comes to saving lives !

You can find her website here : http://gerson.org/gerpress/the-gerson-therapy/

The Budwig Protocol

Dr. Johanna Budwig was a genius and a seven-time alternative Nobel Prize nominee. Dr. Budwig was a qualified pharmacologist, chemist and physicist with a doctorate in physics who worked as the chief expert-consultant for drugs and fats at the former Federal Institute for Fats Research.

Dr. Budwig discovered that healthy people with a normal/healthy pH contained greater levels of Omega 3 essential fatty acids than from blood of someone that was ill.

The Dangers of Hydrogenated Oils

She discovered that most extract the oil for plants, sunflowers, corn, ect by using chemicals and extreme heat, whereby they are no longer alive and are actually dead oils that will cause death to the user. To understand, she explained that they are tough oils meaning dead and that is why they can have a life shelf of over 20 years.

Due to this, these oils get into our cell membranes and destroy the electrical charge. Without this charge our cells will eventually suffocate.

Johanna Budwig successfully helped over 2,400 people with cancer and other illnesses regain their health with her protocol while she was still alive.

The Budwig approach allows you to learn how to treat the cause of many types of cancers including breast cancer, lung cancer, brain cancer, prostate cancer, bone cancer, cervical cancer, stomach cancer, carcinoma, bladder cancer, leukemia, Hodgkin's disease, and skin cancer just to name a few.

Their protocol teaches you how to correct the DNA production cells from bad ones to good ones. When followed correctly they have an 80% to 93% success rate which is unheard of. They even offer a special test which is called the VEGA Testing Device. This will determine if your illness is caused by dental problems, congested liver/gallbladder/kidneys, chemical related, nutritional deficiencies, emotional trauma or hormonal imbalance.

There point is once you learn the cause of your illness you can start treating it appropriately which makes perfect sense.

Now the Budwig Protocol can again either be done at home or you can travel to one of their clinics which offers intensive treatment which some include:

Hyperthermia which creates an artificial fever. Cancer cells cannot withstand heat.

Electro-Magnetic Therapy
Massage Therapy
Lymphatic Drainage
IV Infusions
Ultra Sound Tests
Bio magnetic Therapy
FIR Infrared detox therapy and much more

The Budwig Diet that people use at home is as follows;

Budwig Diet Flaxseed Oil and Cottage Cheese (FOCC) or quark recipe:

Generally, each tablespoon of Flaxseed Oil (FO) is blended with 2 or more tablespoons of low-fat organic Cottage Cheese (CC) or quark.

To make the Budwig Muesli, blend 3 Tablespoons of flaxseed oil (FO) with 6 Tbsp. low-fat(less than 2%) Quark or Cottage Cheese (CC) with a hand-held immersion electric blender for up to a minute.

If the mixture is too thick and/or the oil does not disappear you may need to add 2 or 3 Tablespoons of milk (goat milk would be the best option). Do not add water or juices when blending FO with CC or quark. The mixture should be like rich whipped cream with no separated oil. Remember you must mix ONLY the FO and CC and nothing else at first. Always use organic food products when possible.

Now once the FO and CC are well mixed grind 2 Tbsp. of whole flaxseeds and add to the mixture. Please note that freshly ground flax seeds must be used within 20 minutes after being ground or they will become rancid. Therefore do not grind up flaxseeds ahead of time and store.

Next mix in by hand or with the blender 1 teaspoon of honey (raw non-pasteurized is recommended)

For variety you may add other ingredients such as sugar free apple sauce, cinnamon, vanilla, lemon juice, chopped almonds, hazelnuts, walnuts, cashews (no peanuts), pine kernels, rosehip-marrow. For people who find the Budwig Muesli hard to take these added foods will make the mixture more palatable. Some of our patients have even added a pinch of Celtic sea salt and others put in a pinch of cayenne pepper for a change

(Optional) Add ground up Apricot kernels (no more than 6 kernels per day). Or you may decide to eat these apricot kernels on their own

Nausea - Some people get nausea from the ground flaxseeds, to counter this by taking a small bowl of papaya immediately afterwards. Also put a lot of papaya into the morning muesli too, it may be there is a special enzymes in the papaya that quells the nausea.

The Basic Rule with the Budwig anti-cancer diet is "if God made it then it's fine and try to eat it in the same form that God made it".

Here are some foods that many are not sure of, but they are accepted on the Budwig diet.

Stevia, raw non-pasteurized honey, dates, figs, berry and fruit juices serve as sweeteners.

Herbs in their natural form (pure nothing added)

All nuts (raw unroasted) are fine except peanuts

All seeds good, sunflower seeds are very complete and filling

Raw un processed cocoa, shredded (unsweetened coconut) and rose hip puree

Cup of black tea is accepted (coffee beans are toxic and not recommended)

Any flour is permissible as long as it's 100% whole grain. Corn is generally believed by the group to be an exception because of mold/fungus and genetic manipulation

2 or 3 slices of health food store pickles (no preservatives! - read label!)

Freezing cottage cheese /Quark as well as fruits and vegetables is ok.

VERY IMPORTANT: The flaxseed oil must always be kept in the refrigerator. It will keep for 12 months in the freezer. Arrange to purchase as direct as possible from a manufacturer (like Barlean's) and when it arrives put it right away in the refrigerator. Or arrange with the local health shop to keep a supply in the refrigerator for you.

Drink only distilled water or reverse osmosis water according to Dr. Budwig.

NO hydrogenated oils, NO trans-fats, (all cold pressed oils, such as sunflower seed oil, olive oil, etc)

NO animal fats, NO pork (pigs are the cleaners of the earth and their meat is loaded with toxins. Ham, bacon, sausages, etc should be avoided)

NO seafood (lobsters, clams, shrimp, all fish with a hard shell are cleaners of the sea and are loaded with toxins...)

White regular pasta is eliminated, as is white bread, (Spelt pasta and bread is a better choice than wheat as many cancer patients have an intolerance to wheat, whole Rye, Oat, Multigrain bread is good.

Corn is very discouraged (because of mold and genetic modification issues).

NO ice cream or dairy products (other than the cottage cheese and some cheese)

NO white sugar, molasses, maple syrup or preservatives.

NO processed foods (NO store bought pastries), make your own with the recipes they provide

NO Soy products (unless fermented or used for 2 or 3 weeks at the beginning if you cannot tolerate the cottage cheese)

Avoid pesticides and chemicals, even those in household products & cosmetics. Good old vinegar, as well as baking soda are excellent household cleaners (look on the Internet for more info)

NO microwave, NO Teflon or aluminium cooking ware or aluminium foil. Stainless steel, ceramic, cast iron, glass and corning cooking wear are fine.

Please refer to the site for more information: http://www.budwigcenter.com/anti-cancer-diet.php

Laetril – B17 – Apricot Seeds

Laetrile (Vitamin B17 or amygdalin) is a very popular alternative cancer treatment but is also kept quiet. So popular that one gentleman, Jason Vale used it to cure his cancer, started a website selling the apricot seeds and other items online, but due to advertising them as a **"Cure for Cancer"** on his website he was thrown in jail as these items were alleged as false promises according to the FDA. Vale was released from prison in 2008 and his tumor has come back due to not having access to B17.

Dr. Ernst Krebb, Jr. was the first person to use laetrile in treatments upon his discovery of Vitamin B17 in 1952.

Amygdalin was promoted in a modified form called Laetrile as a cancer cure by Ernst T. Krebs, Jr. under the name "Vitamin B17", but studies have found it to be ineffective and an example of quackery by the FDA and medical world.

Of course they would deem it as quackery! Can you image a cure from buying and eating apricot seeds at such a low cost and again no repeat visits?

Through proven research, a Himalayan tribe known as the Hunza does not have any cases of cancer when consuming their native which includes an exceptionally high consumption of apricots. On a daily basis it is estimated the Hunza consume an average individual ration of between 250 and 3,000 milligrams of vitamin B17.

While we should be jumping for joy with this discovery, it is constantly being supressed by the Big Pharma companies, who are more interested in repeat customers than in curing disease.

Laetrile is a perfectly natural and a safe supplement, although good luck getting your doctor to administer or admit they are using it as the FDA has made the purchase of laetrile supplements close to impossible and if your doctor gets caught using it they will most definately lose their license to practice!

How Laetril/B17 works

When the laetrile compound molecule comes in contact with a cancer cell, it is broken down into 2 molecules of glucose, 1 molecule of hydrogen cyanide and 1 molecule of benzaldehyde.

In the early days of laetrile research it was assumed that the hydrogen cyanide molecule was the major cancer cell killing molecule, but now it is known that it is the benzaldehyde molecule is what kills the cancer cell.

Now I know your thinking oh my god! Cyanide? Cyanide in this form is non-toxic, just like it is in Vitamin B-12.

There is no "free" hydrogen cyanide in Laetrile. When Laetrile comes in contact with the enzyme beta-glucosidase, the Laetrile is broken to form two molecules of glucose, one molecule of benzaldehyde and one molecule of hydrogen cyanide. Within the body, the cancer cell and only the cancer cell contains that enzyme. The word here is that the hydrogen cyanide must be formed. It is not floating around freely in the laetrile and then released.

The enzyme beta glucosidase, and only that enzyme, is capable of manufacturing the hydrogen cyanide from Laetrile. If there are no cancer cells in the body, there is no beta-glucosidase. If there is no beta-blucosidase, no hydrogen cynide will be formed from the Laetrile.

You must understand that Laetrile does contain cyanide. This is the same cyanide radical found in Vitamin B12, in many berry's such as blueberries, blackberries and strawberries. Have you ever heard of anyone getting cyanide poisoning from B12 or of the above berries?

Laetril - B17 - Apricots seeds can help you fight your cancer. There are again hundreds of testimonies to prove it. For more information about Jason Vale and testimonies go here:

http://www.apricotsfromgod.info/

Though it has limitations in certain cancers, vitamin B17 may be extremely effective in the most common tumours such as carcinoma of the lung, breast, prostate, colon, and lymphomas.

A highly publicised clinical trial conducted by the National Cancer Institute in 1981 tried unsuccessfully to prove Laetrile ineffective and toxic. Today, Laetrile occupies a position on the "front lines" of alternative cancer therapy.

"We have found Laetrile to be effective in people that have active cancer", says Dr. Contreras "but that is not its only function, for the prevention of cancer and the maintenance of remission there is nothing as effective as Laetrile. Its non-toxicity permits its use indefinitely in the prevention of relapses and the prevention of metastases. Surgery, radiation, and chemotherapy can only be administered for a limited time afterward patients are left without any protection".

For a more detailed analysis of the theoretical action of Laetrile against cancer cells, see G. Edward Griffin which can be found on the internet.

"A control for cancer is known, and it comes from nature, but it is not widely available to the public because it cannot be patented, and therefore is not commercially attractive to the pharmaceutical industry."
-G. Edward Griffin

Intravenous Vitamin C

Thirty years ago Cameron, Campbell and Pauling's reported beneficial effects of high-dose vitamin C (absorbic acid) therapy for patients with terminal cancer. Subsequent double-blind, randomized clinical trials at the Mayo Clinic failed to show any benefit, and the role of vitamin C in cancer treatment was discarded by mainstream oncologists.

Nothing new here... Again you must understand there is no money to be made, no repeat customers and no patents, so they will discard it!

However, vitamin C continues to be used successfully as an alternative for cancer therapy still to this day.

Irwin Stone was the early writer about vitamin C and understood it would be a challenge to get the medical world to view vitamin C in a different light. Most doctors accept and now understand that Vitamin C was the deficiency that caused Scurvy and killed so many, however few have made the acceptance that seeing high dose intravenous vitamin C as a major player in the management of cancer.

Dr. Huge Riordan checked plasma vitamin C levels in chronically ill patients and found them to be consistently low in vitamin C levels. Cancer patients had extremely low reserves of vitamin C.

When large amounts of vitamin C are introduced to cancer cells they will be absorbed in those large amounts. In these large amounts the antioxidant vitamin C will start acting as a pro-oxidant.

This chemical interaction produces small amounts of hydrogen peroxide.

Due to cancer cells being low in intracellular anti-oxidant enzyme called catalase, the high dose vitamin C induction of peroxide will continue to build up until it eventually breaks down the cell from the inside out and destroy it.

This essentially and effectively makes high dose Intravenous vitamin C a non-toxic chemotherapy agent that can be given with other conventional or alternative cancer treatments.

Based on the work of several vitamin C pioneers, Dr. Riordan was able to prove that vitamin C was selectively toxic to cancer cells if given intravenously.

Intravenous vitamin C also does more than just kill cancer cells. It boosts the immunity of the ill individual which is the most important factor to a cancer patient.

The first ever study in which vitamin C was given to cancer patients was carried out in the 1970s, by Dr. Linus Pauling and Dr. Ewan Cameron, cancer specialists, working in Scotland. They gave 100 terminally ill cancer patients 10g (10,000mg) of vitamin C each day and compared their outcome with 1000 cancer patients given conventional therapy.

The survival rate was five times higher in those taking vitamin C. By 1978, while all of the 1000 'control patients' had died, 13 of the vitamin C patients were still alive, with 12 apparently free from cancer. Other studies have confirmed these findings.

Dr Murata and Dr Morishige of Saga University in Japan showed that cancer patients on 5–30g of vitamin C lived six times longer than those on 4g or less, while those suffering from cancer of the uterus lived 15 times longer on vitamin C therapy. This was also confirmed by the late Dr. Abram Hoffer in Canada, who found that patients on high doses of vitamin C survived, on average, ten times longer.

However, vitamin C for cancer suffered a major setback when Dr. Charles Moertel of the Mayo Clinic sought to disprove Pauling's thesis on the theory of vitamin C treatment for cancer. But he did not follow the Pauling/Cameron instructions or regimen which ultimately skewed the data.

There are many clinics and doctors that successfully use and treat cancer with intravenous vitamin C.

There are many that will tell you many set backs about using vitamin C, especially your oncologist. I know when I spoke to my father's onocologist about this topic and other alternative therapy's he just dismissed them.

I urge you to do your research and thoroughly invegstigate the topic further. Many cancer survivors have used this therapy in conjunction with many of the others listed in this book.

The Power of Barley Leaves Extracts

I discovered Bob Davis's website in late February 2013 and was amazed by his story. I had never heard of this powerful little product by nature and am estatic to have stumbled upon it it.

He is 91 and has beat cancer twice!

Here is Bob's story in his words:

In April 1996, I was admitted to the hospital as an outpatient for an x-ray. It was found that I had massive cancer. I had a mass in my abdomen a foot wide and several inches thick. Further, I had several masses in my chest, some of them "the size of soft balls". It was also determined that I had cancer in my bone marrow.

I was immediately converted into an "in" patient and started on a very heavy chemotherapy program. I had chemo in April, May, and June, with no effect on the cancer. It seemed to thrive on the stuff.

It was the middle of June when my doctor told me that the chemo wasn't working. He later told me that another treatment would kill me. I knew that this was true because my body was ravaged by the chemo. I was curled up in a fetal position unable to sleep or eat. I was emaciated and had excruciating pain all through my body.

I asked my doctor what we were going to do. He said, "Try..........something else"

The previous February I had called a college chum who had devastating arthritis. He couldn't climb stairs or drive his car. I asked him how he was doing and he said "Fantastic"! He told me that he was taking an herbal product and it had eliminated his arthritis in three weeks. I asked him what it was and he said "Dried green barley leaves". He gave me the 800 number and I ordered a bottle for my wife who has arthritis.

It was the middle of June as I mention above, that I received a phone call from the owner of the company that provides the dried green barley pills. She asked me how I was doing on the pills. I told her that I wasn't using them. I had gotten them for my wife and they helped her when she remembered to take them.

I then said the most fortunate thing I have said in my life. I said, "I'm fighting another battle". She asked me what it was and I told her that it was cancer. She said, "Oh, Mr. Davis, You don't know do you"? I asked her what was it that I didn't know and she said, "Don't you know that cancer and arthritis can't grow in an alkaline body"? I told her that I had never heard that before.

To make a long story short (one of my favorite phrases), I started taking the pills and in ten days my cancer was 95% gone! My next Ct scan showed no cancer in my body and I have been cancer free ever since.

I was checked last month and I am still cancer free. I still take 20 200 mg tablets of dried green barley every day. It costs me a whopping 95 cents or so.

What is Barley Leaves Extract?

For one it's delicious, green powder, revolutionary and most importantly packed with all the essential vitamins, minerals, enzymes, chlorophyll, and antioxidants in a naturally balanced form.

The amazing power of young barley leaves helps you restore your body pH easily.

Barley Leaves Extract helps fight:

- High blood pressure
- High cholesterol
- Heart disease
- Cancer
- Diabetes
- Liver problems
- AIDS
- Allergies
- Body odor
- Aging
- Wrinkles and tired skin
- Free radical formation just to name a few

How Barley Leaves Extract Fight Cancer

The barley leaves extract contains an enzyme known as peroxidase. This enzyme makes carcinogenic substances harmless and prevents normal cells from becoming cancerous.

They also contain a large amount of antioxidant vitamin A, C, and E, which supress carcinogenic substances. Since these vitamins work together in Barley Leaves Extract, it is entirely possible that they might be more effective in conquering cancer than when used individually.

Barley Leaves contain Vital Vitamins

They are the complete source of vitamins in its natural form. Barley Leaves Extract contains an amazing number of vitamins, such as carotenoids (which convert to vitamin A), vitamins B1, B2, B6, C, E, niacin, choline, biotin, and essential amino acids.

Trace Elements and Minerals

Principle minerals and numerous trace elements work hand in hand with vitamins for a balanced body. Without minerals, no living creature could function properly.

Minerals are metallic elements which we would recognize as iron, potassium, copper, zinc, and manganese. These are just a few.

The human body requires only a tiny amount of these minerals, although a deficiency in these minerals can result in a myriad of serious diseases. Also many enzymes cannot function properly without minerals.

The wonderful thing about Barley Leaves Extracts is they contain a huge amount of minerals which is perfect to create a balanced body.

Activate and energize with enzymes

Our bodies need enzymes to function properly. There has been more than 3,000 enzymes identified in the human body and they all work in different ways. Barley Leaves Extract contains hundreds of essential live enzymes to facilitate vital body functions.

Barley Leaves Extract is an alkaline/acid balancer which is so often lacking in most western diets. Barley is one of the most alkaline foods known to man. Because of the natural calcium, beta carotene, protein, iron, other vitamins and minerals, plus live enzymes, this aids the body to either return to an alkaline state or continue to stay in an alkaline state, which is vitally essential!

The point to take away is that Green Barely Leave Extract builds the immune system on a cellular level and balances your body's pH levels which are critical for a healthy body.

I know many that have added Barley Leaves Extract into their protocols. Some do 5 to 9 different protocols together at once.

I personally take 10 barley leaf pills per day and will continue for the rest of my life!

The Power of Essential Oils

Here is another truly amazing natural substance from nature that has remarkable healing powers. The two I would like to discuss are Orange and Frankincense oils.

I stumbled upon Irene and Walter Tomaszewsky's website a few months back. Another amazing natural healing story about Walter and him becoming Cancer free after his wife took matters into her own hands.

Walter was diagnosed with non-Hodgkin's mantle cell lymphoma in November of 2011. He is now cancer free as of January 2013.

You can find her website here: http://transform-yourhealth.com/

The Power of Orange Essential Oil

Essential oils from the orange tree's flowers, leaves, and rind have powerfully healing effects. Amazingly anti-carcinogenic and anti-tumoral based on its high 85%-96% limonene chemistry; this oil has combated tumor growth in over 50 clinic studies.

Source: Essential Oils for Physical Health & Well-Being by Linda L. Smith

Clinical trials using d-limonene as a cancer inhibitor have been conducted for well over a decade. D-Limonene and its digestion by-product Perillyl alcohol have been studied at the University of Wisconsin, Indiana University-Purdue University, with a new JAN 2010 clinical trial taking form at the University of Arizona as well as various medical center trials.

Now why is this not widely spread in medical journals or in fact just common knowledge?

The unfortunate fact is that most doctors and oncologists are not taught about this or are not aware of Perillyl alcohol's and D-Limonene's benefits or more so there just isn't enough financial incentive to have cancer patients self-administer orange oil for their own natural cancer recovery.

June 1997 ~ Cancer Chemoprevention and Therapy by Monoterpenes by M N Gould, Department of Human Oncology, University of Wisconsin, Madison USA

"Monoterpenes are found in the essential oils of many plants including fruits, vegetables, and herbs. They prevent the carcinogenesis process at both the initiation and promotion/progression stages. In addition, monoterpenes are effective in treating early and advanced cancers.

Monoterpenes such as limonene and perillyl alcohol have been shown to prevent mammary, liver, lung, and other cancers. These compounds have also been used to treat a variety of rodent cancers, including breast and pancreatic carcinomas. In addition, in vitro data suggest that they may be effective in treating neuroblastomas and leukemia's."

Another interesting article by Mark Brudnak PhD, ND is a board certified naturopath. He states the following:

Dr. Brudnak writes "While the MTs [monoterpenes] are indeed used as cleaning (try placing a small amount on the front hubcaps of your car to clean off the black grime) agents, due to their solvent properties, they are far from being poisons. Indeed, nothing could be further from the truth for these wonderful, naturally occurring, and health-promoting substances. While the solvent properties of monoterpenes have been exploited clinically to dissolve gallstones, the monoterpenes are also the focus of much investigation in the area of cancer prevention and therapeutics…

Cancer prevention, inhibition, and regression are the most noteworthy attributes of the MTs (monoterpenes).

D-limonene (DL) and perillyl alcohol (POH) have been shown to be chemo-preventive against mammary, liver, lung, UV-induced skin cancers, and chemotherapeutic against both experimental mammary and pancreatic tumours. Perillyl alcohol stands out as effective against human pancreatic cancer, colon, liver cancers, to reduce vein graft intimal hyperplasia, as chemo-preventive against colon carcinogenesis, prostate and lung cancers.

Personal Orange Oil Anti-Cancer Testimonials are popping up everywhere!

Vicki Opfer's Young Living group in Arvada, CO reports ORANGE therapeutic-quality essential oil is demonstrating great promise against cancer…helping the body rid itself of cancer. When people are willing to ingest 10ml of orange oil (in capsules) every day, and it is a lot of Orange essential oil - 2/3 of a 15ml bottle daily, this replicates the amount of limonene in studies which have demonstrated a regression of cancer.

She continues to write:

~ While in Japan recently, a woman of about 45 shared she had been told last summer 2009 her uterine cancer had spread throughout her body and she only had a month to live. The doctors said , due to her condition they were not able to offer surgery or chemotherapy. After speaking with a Young Living leader there, she took 10ml of orange oil every day, in capsules. She also rubbed the therapeutic-quality orange oil, frankincense, myrtle, sandalwood, and tsuga essential oils all over her belly every day, and drank 4-6 oz. NingXia Red (nutritional juice) each day, as well. She is now CANCER FREE!

~ From C.D. in New Jersey: "My mother-in-law had a grapefruit-sized tumor on her only remaining kidney. Her other kidney had been destroyed by cancer 5 years earlier. The doctors could not treat her because of her deteriorating health, so she began to take 10 ml of orange oil in capsules. She took 2 full capsules every 2 hours for eight hours a day. After 3 months the tumor was gone. She continues to take 1-4 capsules of orange oil and also drinks 2-4 oz. Ningxia Red every day. Her CANCER has NOT returned."

SOURCE: April 2010 ISHA Aromatherapy Newsletter

One important factor to note is that all citrus essential oils have compounds that may cause sunburn / skin damage with sun exposure. When your applying the citrus oils topically, you should not be exposing yourself to the sun or at least cover up. You should stay out of the sun for 12 hours after an application.

Irene started her husband Walter on Orange and Frankincense oil internally. Within 5 weeks, his blood tests revealed a significant improvement. He would take 200 drops of orange oil and 60 drops of frankincense oil internally, as well as having them rubbed on his skin of the affected area.

The Power of Frankincense Oil

Scientists have observed that there is some agent within frankincense which stops cancer spreading, and which induces cancerous cells to close themselves down. He is trying to find out what this is.

Here's an excerpt: Immunologist Mahmoud Suhail is hoping to open a new chapter in the history of frankincense…

"Cancer starts when the DNA code within the cell's nucleus becomes corrupted," he says. "It seems frankincense has a re-set function. It can tell the cell what the right DNA code should be.

"Frankincense separates the 'brain' of the cancerous cell – the nucleus – from the 'body' – the cytoplasm, and closes down the nucleus to stop it reproducing corrupted DNA codes."

Working with frankincense could revolutionise the treatment of cancer. Currently, with chemotherapy, doctors blast the area around a tumour to kill the cancer, but that also kills healthy cells, and weakens the patient. Treatment with frankincense could eradicate the cancerous cells alone and let the others live.

SOURCE:http://news.bbc.co.uk/1/hi/world/middle_east/8505251.stm

Dr. Suhail, which works in Oman as a physician stated that they can't do clinical cancer research there because nobody in Oman has cancer. There are NO cancer units at the two hospitals there.

He sees 1 or 2 people with cancer every couple of years and I think he said those are people who have lived outside the country.

The local people chew the frankincense resin and also soak it overnight and drink the water, so it is very much a part of their lives.

Here is an amazing article that you may want to read at a later date: http://news.bbc.co.uk/2/hi/middle_east/8505251.stm

PROPERTIES: Anti-Catarrhal, Anti-Depressant, Anti-Infectious, Anti-Inflammatory, Antiseptic, Anti-Tumoral, Expectorant, Immune-stimulant (increases leukocyte activity to defend the body against infection), supports Nerves, prevents Scarring, Sedative.

BODY SYSTEM(S) AFFECTED:

Emotionally: Frankincense promotes acceptance, emotional balance & stability, offers protection, fortitude, courage & resolution; increases introspection, spiritual awareness & inspiration, is an aid in meditative practices & prayer work.

Physically: Frankincense supports the immune, bronchial, cardiovascular, digestive systems; nerves; skin, and is protective against many ailments & diseases such as diphtheria, gonorrhea, jaundice, herpes, meningitis, syphilis, TB, typhoid.

Immune Boosters

If you have a strong immune system, the fact is that you are healthy and strong. You will not see cancer grow or thrive in the body of a person that has a strong immune system because they have a balanced pH level.

Our body's ability to fight off disease is due to our incredible immune system. For cancer to develop, your immune system must either be ineffective, worn out or unable to kill cancer cells as fast as they develop.

Bottom line, it is vital to restore and strengthen your immune system in order to win your battle against cancer.

I had read an article on Dr. Matthias, who did research based on Dr. Linus Pauling's earlier work and as he indicated as an opener to precursory treatment to any chronic condition is based on 3 vitamins and amino acids which are:

1. Vitamin C (preferably fat - soluble, aka ascorbyl palmitate)
2. L-Lysine
3. L- Proline

On his site: http://www.probiotics-for-health.com/cure-protocols.html scroll down to the links and click on cancer. This pdf report explains in depth and helps you understand how cells move through the body, natural enzyme block, enzyme blocks in cancer therapy, how cancer spreads and so much more. It is very important for you to understand this if you or a loved one have cancer.

The main Immune Booster supplement that one should be on if stricken with cancer is the following:

Heart Plus Veg Caps

Supplemental Facts
Vitamin C - 500mg

L-Lysine - 500mg
L-Proline - 200mg
Rose Hips - 50 mg

You can find them here: http://ourhealthcoop.com/

The other is Beta 1, 3d Glucan:

You can find them here: http://www.ancient5.com/Transfer-Point-Beta-Glucan-500mg-p/tpbg-500-60.htm

How Beta Glucan Helps the Immune System Fight Cancer

According to Dr. Vetvicka at the School of Medicine in Louisville, Kentucky, beta glucan stimulates the immune system and helps fight invading tumor cells. Stress, allergies, pollutants and age compromise the immune system leaving it in need of help. This is where beta glucan comes in. Under normal conditions, the immune system is able to overcome the invasion of cancer cells, but when it is compromised, the defense is weakened against the development of tumors.

Scientific literature purports that even a healthy immune system cannot adequately deal with fast-growing cancer cells alone. Beta glucan can assist the immune system in destroying only the cancer cells leaving the surrounding tissues and organs intact and unharmed. Compared to traditional treatment of cancer, beta glucan treatment has one big advantage – no negative side effects to date.

How Beta Glucan works as stated on Ancient 5 website:

While simple sugars would be broken down in the digestive system, converting into glucose for energy use, this does not occur with a complex carbohydrate fiber like Beta Glucan.

Beta 1, 3-D glucan works by activating immune cells known as macrophages (neutrophils and natural killer (NK) cells.) These are your immune system's first line of innate defense.

They are responsible for finding, identifying and consuming foreign substances in the body. Macrophages also control the activities of other important cells in the immune system. "Because macrophages can be found in almost every organ of our body, including the brain, they are in an ideal position to react." says Dr. Vaclav Vetvicka.

Beta glucan has been proven to be effective when administered orally and intravenously; however, the latter would require daily visits to a physician. When taken orally, the macrophage obtains maximum activity and effectiveness after about 72 hours, then again reaches normal activity after about 144 hours.

This polysaccharide is carried across the lining of the small intestine into the lymphatic system via M (microfold) cells in the Peyer's Patches. From the lymphatic system, the Beta Glucan is carried by phagocytes throughout the immune system and bone marrow. This provides complete systemic activation of your immune system.

When you're battling cancer you have no time to waste at all. You have to act as quickly as possible and your first step should be to boost your immune system as fast as you can!

Diet, Nutrition & Detox

Today, many are finally realizing that diet is tied to so many diseases of all types. Treatment using a raw diet is absolutely mandatory as the majority of patients are not getting well with the standard western medicine and oncology that is being offered today.

You must understand that in today's society the majority of our meals are processed, overcooked and full of pesticides, herbicides and fungicides. Our water is polluted with fluoride and purified with chlorine. One of the by-products from using chloride in our drinking water is linked to cancer.

When you are battling cancer you have to change your diet to a healthy one as fast as you can. Yes, it's hard but if it means saving your life, it's well worth the change.

Knowing and understanding which foods feed the cancer cells, which ones interfere with treatment and the one's that assist with natural healing are essential to one's battle.

All natural plant foods contain nutrients that aid in healing the body at the cellular level. Fruits, vegetables and herbs have certain properties that inhibit the growth of cancer and protect the body while strengthening and repairing it at the same time.

It's a known fact to many that we are overloaded with Omega 6's and deficient in Omega 3's.

Any cancer patient should aim for a diet that is 80% raw. This will ensure that they are consuming an alkaline diet, an abundance of enzymes which aid in the healing process. Also oral supplementation of digestive enzymes with meals will also further aid in healing naturally.

Pancreative enzymes digest away the protein wall or coating which protects the cancer cell from being destroyed by the immune system, aka, our natural killer cells.

Why Juice?

In today's society people are becoming more aware of the importance of juicing. We are nutritionally deprived at a cellular level.

It is a fact that cooking and processing foods destroy essential micro-nutrients by altering their shape and chemical compositions. All enzymes are lost when you cook any food. Our bodies then have to manufacture its own enzymes to do the work because our body recognizes these overcooked and processed foods as a foreign substance.

By juicing, the body does not have to work overtime to produce enzymes that are needed to transform cooked food into usable nutrients for cellular regeneration. It has been stated over and over again by the medical authority's that we need at least 6-8 servings of fruits and vegetables per day. How many servings are you getting?

Really think about that.

The majority of us don't even come close to this amount due to our busy and hectic schedules. Juicing is a simple way to absolutely guarantee that you will reach your daily servings without any problems.

When you drink fresh juices, the cells are flooded with life giving nutrients. The important ingredients from juicing with raw foods are the active enzymes that your body uses to transform nutrients into a usable form for cellular health and growth. Nutrients from the fresh juices get to the cells and are absorbed in the bloodstream within a few minutes.

Another factor about juicing is your eliminating the harmful sprays and pesticides if you're not organically growing it yourself.

Top 3 Benefits to Juicing

Weight Loss
Increased Energy
Immune Booster

You can easily get your intake of your vegetables and fruits without feeling very full. It allows you to absorb all the essentials nutrients with less digestion. Due to poor food choices many of us have compromised our digestion systems, which limit our ability to absorb all the appropriate nutrients from the veggies we eat.

Again, think of the nutrients being delivered straight to your cells, which give your digestion system a break. This is an incredible way to boost your immune system. You're giving your body on a cellular level a huge mega dose of the nutrients which in turn will strengthen your immune system and give you more energy.

There have been countless of success stories that have kicked cancer in the arse just by changing their diet to an alkaline one, by juicing and detoxing. Again when you do this, you are flooding your body on a cellular level a massive amount of nutrients, vitamins and enzymes that are needed to build up the immune systems (aka. Killer cells) to fight your cancer battle.

Why Detox, Specifically Coffee Enemas?

When you are battling cancer either naturally or traditionally your cancer cells will start to die off. These dead cells have to go somewhere which are dying off in large quantities. They have to be expelled.

Cancer patients normally have a body full of toxic substances; this is normally the main cause of the cancer in the first place. These toxins must be flushed out of the cells and organs, and are required to be expelled out of the body as quickly as possible.

While treating your cancer, if this is not done, the individual may experience an overflow of toxins into the liver, and can cause organ malfunction due to the overburden of the toxins to your organs.

Coffee enemas date back to 1914 during World War I. During that time, morphine was no longer available but the wounded soldiers from battle kept on arriving at the hospitals.

It's explained that when the doctors finished operating, they would order plain water enemas for their patients but the nurses were desperately looking for something else to ease the pain for these soldiers.

One of the nurses decided to try the left over coffee that the surgeons drank. Amazingly the wounded soldiers reported that their pain started to diminish.

Peter Lechner M.D., an oncologist surgeon did coffee enemas for his patients for 6 years under a controlled testing environment. Independent laboratory results proved that Coffee Enemas played a major role in detoxifying the liver and assisting in the recovery of the patients.

Understand that when you're killing off cancer cells at a fast rate you must expel the waste just as quickly. Your liver is the body's filtration system and coffee enemas have proven themselves as a means to restore the liver to an optimum state.

How it works:

While you are holding the coffee enema in the gut for a period of 12 to 15 minutes, all of your body's blood is being passed through the liver every 3 minutes. Due to the solution being coffee and not saline water it allows the blood vessels to dilate and the liver's portal veins to dilate as well. Due to this, the bile ducts expand with blood, the bile flow starts to increase and the internal organs relax.

Holding the coffee enema for 12 to 15 minutes means that your blood just went through your liver about 5 times! Massive detoxification!

As stated by Dr. Peter Lechner, it lowers the quantity of blood serum toxins, literally cleaning the poisons out of fluids while nourishing normal cells.

The other important role of using coffee is that it stimulates the increase of the production of Glutathione S- Transferase (GST) by 600-700%. This GST is an enzyme that contributes to the removal of free radicals and toxins from the blood. The radicals and toxins then leave the liver and gallbladder as bile salts flowing through the duodenum. Essentially these are then carried out by peristalsis action which travels from the small intestine, to the colon and out of the rectum.

Jess Ainscough fought and beat cancer utilizing the Gerson Therapy and employing coffee enemas on a regular basis. She has an amazing video that shows you in depth on how to perform them if you're interested in learning more.

http://www.thewellnesswarrior.com.au/2011/11/wellness-warrior-tv-how-to-do-a-coffee-enema/

Coffee enemas can relieve the patient of depression, the body's toxins, confusion, allergy-related symptoms and most importantly severe pain.

Essiac Tea

Essiac name was first given by Rene Caisse ("caisse" spelt backwards), and this powerhouse tea consist of four main herbs that grow in Canada.

The original formula is believed to originate from the Ojibway Indians native to Canada. These herbs are Sheep Sorrel, Indian Rhubarb Root, Burdock Root and Slippery Elm Inner Bar.

Essiac Tea dates back to the 1920's and has been an old proven method of curing cancer.

Caisse theorized that one of the herbs in Essiac reduced tumor growth while the others acted as blood purifiers which will elimate destroyed tissue as well as infections which were a result of the malignancy. The main herb to be known as the cancer killeris Sheep Sorrel.

Main Benefits:

Restoring the Immune System

By cleaning your body of toxins this frees up the immune system to focus on killing cancer cells and protect the body. Drinking Essiac Tea allows for a complete body purifcation to happen, which allows a large boost in your's body immune system to fight any pre-existing disease by producing more lymphocytes and T-cells which are the bodys natural defenses.

Detoxification:

Essiac tea aids the body to release toxins that build up in the fat and tissues in the blood stream whereby they can be filtered and expelled by the liver and kidneys. Eliminating these toxins is critical in your fight against cancer and cancer cell growth. It also aids your organs and immune system and helps it to run at an optimum level.

How does the tea work?

Cancer patients normally have a compromised immune system which lowers their natural bodys defenses. Essiac tea aids to help cleanse the body of toxins while repairing the immune system and strengthen your vital organs. As a result, this allows your body to fight as it should at an optimum level.

Essiac Tea has a natural source of vitamins, minerals which all contain antioxidants which are known to protect against cellular damage caused by free radicals.

The Formula:

The following formula and recipe for Essiac (in italics) is a word-for-word transcription of the Essiac formula from the sworn affidavit which Mary McPherson filed with the Town of Bracebridge.

6 ½ cups of burdock root (cut)
1 pound of sheep sorrel herb powdered
1/4 pound of slippery elm bark powdered
1 ounce of Turkish rhubarb root powdered

Mix these ingredients thoroughly and store in glass jar in dark dry cupboard.

Take a measuring cup, use 1 ounce of herb mixture to 32 ounces of water depending on the amount you want to make.

I use 1 cup of mixture to 8 x 32 = 256 ounces of water. Boil hard for 10 minutes (covered) then turn off heat but leave sitting on warm plate overnight (covered).

In the morning heat steaming hot and let settle a few minutes, then strain through fine strainer into hot sterilized bottles and sit to cool. Store in dark cool cupboard. Must be refrigerated when opened. When near the last when its thick pour in a large jar and sit in frig overnight then pour off all you [can] without sediment.

This recipe must be followed exactly as written.

Use a granite preserving kettle (10 – 12 qts), 8 ounce measuring cup, small funnel and fine strainer to fill bottles.

[Here is a detailed video on how to make essiac tea at home.](#)

[Here is also a reliable site that you may purchase at.](#)

Many have combined Essiac Tea with many different protocols.

Testing

You can be pro-active and start checking yourself for cancer at your own expense and convenience.

Upon many phone conversations with Colleen (whom beat breast cancer) told me about this test to check my father's cancer markers. She explained that you do not need a doctor's prescription in order to have it done.

You do the procedure in the comfort of your home and then send it off to this specific clinic in the Philippines. This is one of the most accurate screenings with a track record of over 80 years to determine the level of "abnormally dividing cells" within your body.

This test is called the HCG Test. It was developed in the late 1950's, by the renowned oncologist, the late Dr. Manuel D. Navarro.

The test detects the presence of cancer cells even before signs or symptoms develop.

In short, the test is based on a theory proposed by Howard Beard and a few other researchers who concluded that cancer is related to a misplaced trophoblastic cell that becomes malignant in a manner similar to pregnancy in that they both secrete HCG. The amount of HCG found in the blood or urine is also a measure of the degree of malignancy. The higher the number, the greater cancer is present within the body.

As per Navarro medical clinic's website and numerous other online resources, Navarro test detects the presence of brain cancer as early as 29 months before symptoms appear, 27 months for fibro sarcoma of the abdomen, 24 months for skin cancer and 12 months for cancer of the bones. Currently, many cancer patients take advantage of the diagnostic accuracy of this test as an indicator of the effectiveness of their specific mode of therapy.

Patients follow simple directions for preparing a dry extract from the urine sample. This powdery extract is mailed to the Navarro Medical Clinic in Philippines where the HCG testing is performed.

A test score of 50 (that is 50mIU/ml) or above, means, you probably have cancer. While a score below 50, means, you likely do not have cancer. Thus, if your first test score was 52.7 and second test score is 51.5, your alternative cancer treatment is most likely working. However, if your first test score was 52.7 and second score is 53.9, you might want to look at other treatment options.

You can find there website here:
http://www.navarromedicalclinic.com/index.php

Cancer patients use the Navarro test score to measure the effectiveness of their treatment. But people without cancer can take Navarro test to get an early warning or, just have peace of mind.

The Reality of Western Medicine

At McGill Cancer Center there was a poll taken by accredited scientists which included 118 doctors who are all considered experts on cancer.

If these doctors were to be stricken with cancer, they were asked which "experimental" therapy they would choose from. 3 out of 4 denied all chemotherapy choices due to its devastating effects on the immune system and body and of course the low success rate. They also concluded they would not allow their family members to go through the process either.

So please explain to me and the public and help me understand why almost 75% of doctors we put our trust into are still recommending chemotherapy to their patients when they themselves won't touch it with a 10 foot pole?

Maybe it's that large price tag associated with it when they are recommending it?

Below are a just a few FDA approved chemotherapy drugs and some sickening side effects. I only listed a few as there are too many to list here and I am not even going to cover Radiation Therapy.

Temodar (temozolomide) Chemotherapy

Side Effects:

Hair loss, constipation, nausea and vomiting can be quite severe.

Decreased blood cells.

Temodar affects cells that group rapidly, including bone marrow cells. This can cause you to have a decrease in blood cells. White blood cells are needed to fight infection. Neutrophils are a type of white blood cell that helps prevent bacterial infections. Decreased neutrophils can lead to serious infections that can lead to death.

Source: http://www.merck.com/product/usa/pi_circulars/t/temodar_capsules/temodar_ppi.pdf

Mitotane Chemotherapy

Appropriate studies have not been performed to find out mitotaines safety or effectiveness in children. Source: The Mayo Clinic, 2010

Side Effects:

Nausea, vomiting, depression, changes in vision, rash or changes in skin color, feeling that the room is spinning, abdominal or side pain, fast heartbeat, high fever or shaking chills, excessive sweating.

Mitotane may cause brain or nervous system damage.

Source: http://www.nlm.nih.gov/medlineplus/druginfo/meds/a608050.html#side-effects

Doxorubicin Chemotherapy

Side Effects:

Leukemia, heart failure, infertility, vomiting, mouth sores

Nickname: Red Death

Source: American Cancer Society 2010 (cancer.org)
How Doctors Think, J. Groopman, 2007 p49

Etoposide Chemotherapy

Side Effects:

Leukemia, Nerve damage, inability to fight infections, vomiting.

Source: American Cancer Society 2010 (cancer.org)

Cisplatin Chemotherapy

Side Effects:

Kidney damage, hearing damage, nerve damage, infertility, vomiting.

Source: American Cancer Society 2010 (cancer.org)

You must understand that chemotherapy drugs are such toxic and dangerous substances that if a spill occurs in a hospital, it is considered a major biohazard.

Here is a document on pages 3 and 4 just how much of a big deal a chemo spill is: http://www.utoledo.edu/depts/safety/docs/HM-08-013.pdf

The main foundation of today's Western Medicine is supported by a common saying, ***"A pill for every ill."*** This statement is so far from being correct, it's not funny.

It's supported by radiation treatments, chemotherapy and prescription medication like a child going to the candy store. The main important factor to keep in mind are that these forms of "medicine" are very expensive, patentable, and manipulated by the FDA, Government, media advertising, and Big Pharma.

For decades we have been coerced into making choices of which type of toxin should we be taking as they are highly recommended from the doctors we put our faith and trust into, and then of course all forms of natural healing have either been labeled as "quackery" or *risky* alternative therapy.

Right now the government we trust whether it be the United States, Canada, Australia or any country, they are making sure that the public are consuming foods which absolutely <u>DO</u> cause disease and then receive toxic chemicals as there so called "cures."

This is not good intention or accidental and if you think it is, then you need to really take a second look at what is going on. Remember the term, "Think Tank?" Well that is the fiasco that is going on amongst our political, economic and financial US politicians and money driven scientists.

As stated earlier, Cancer treatment alone is a 300 billion dollar industry. The National Cancer Institute (NCI), the American Cancer Society (ACS), and the Food and Drug Administration (FDA) are the head mob when it comes to their publishing misguided information for the AMA'S (American Medical Association) JAMA (Journal of the American Medical Association), which is the "prestigious" journal whereby Western doctors cling to for drug deals, which inturn make all their patients into "clients for life."

Fact: *Many of the Nazi scientists that served a 4 to 7 year term for mass murder just after World War II, were released from prison and employed by the U.S. corporations to construct a slow death food and medicine for the United States' chronic care management agenda.*

So what is this so called "think tank" agenda behind devising such a plan? Well of course feed the population with unlabeled GMO pesticide corn and soy, aspartame, dump fluoride in our water systems, pump up our animals with antibiotic and hormones, oh and don't forget about the yummy fructose corn syrup (HFCS) we consume regularly.

Then the planned choice of action when sickness prevails is: chemotherapy, pharmaceutical drugs and radiation, and of course surgery. This is not coincidence. It's planned and planned well.

After watching the movie, "Food Matters" it made me realize that when you donate money for an actual cure, these funds are actually spent shutting down the actual cure.

What you must understand is that half the ACS board consists of oncologists and radiologists which are interested in 4 slow death choices for patient. They all receive grants from one another which conclude the circle of trust with cancer funding and that it will keep going round in the same trusted circle.

When you donate money the ACS has whistle blowers for the doctors that are prescribing "unproven methods" , such as natural cures, and then these doctors are shut down in courts and some thrown in jail or their license taken away.

When you find a protocol, therapy, or cure that is cheap, has no side effects or is not patentable, it gets shut down immediately. The AMA is responsible for licensing all doctors in America, so their partners in crime such as the FDA, ACS and NCI serve as the police for identifying doctors that step out of line (meaning: stumbling upon natural cures and letting the public know).

One of the mainstream problems that have been going on for decades is the fact that when a natural cure has been found by an accredited doctor it is then taken by the AMA and the FDA to manipulate and dilute the formulas, so they can post clinical trials showing that the cure "doesn't work."

This is exactly what they did to Dr. Burzynski. He is one doctor that has fought hard to prove that there is a cure. He was not afraid to go against the Big Pharma to prove it and his cancer survivors even stood up in court to defend him. He cured 100's of patients.
The video is an amazing watch and I encourage you to take the time to educate yourself a little further into exactly what is going on with the corruption when it comes to "Cancer Wars."

He was also able to reveal and prove the fabricated FDA research where he discovered and revealed they had diluted his formula intentionally so it would fail and be recorded within the medical journals as a non-curable drug.

Here is a video that is a must watch for everyone: http://vimeo.com/24821365

Here is another major issue that just happened in Ontario, Canada:

Just recently in Ontrario, Canada, is what health officials are calling one of the worst medication errors they've ever seen. Nearly 1,000 cancer patients who received diluted chemotherapy drugs during the course of their treatment. DILUTED!!!

In Windsor, a $25-million notice of class-action lawsuit was filed with the court against the drug supplier.

People are starting to wake up and realize that there needs to be a change and it's need to be now, not later. When you hear the ads stating, "We are close to a cure, or 5 more years," that is such a misconception and will never happen.

It's too the point now that we have to educate ourselves and not just rely on the medical professional as our educator.

"Cancer therapy is so toxic and dehumanizing that I fear it far more than I fear death from cancer itself." -Ralph W.Moss, Ph.D.

Sources:
http://www.drheise.com/chemotherapy.htm
http://www.mnwelldir.org/docs/cancer1/altthrpy.htm
http://www.sntp.net/fda/ama_lynes.htm

Other Protocols & Links

As stated previously, I think there is close to over 350 different protocols to date.

Here are a list of just a few others that you can investigate:

The Photon Protocol
Cellect-Budwig
Bob Wright Protocol
Skilling-Kehr
Plasma Beck
Life One
Rife-Beck
Organic Sulfur Protocol
Overnight Cure for Cancer
Grape Cure
Ozone RHP
Alternative Cancer Clinics
Cesium Chloride
Supplement Treatments
Kelmum Protocol
Hydrogen Peroxide
Hemp Oil
Raw Food Diet
Essiac Tea
Wheat Grass
Noni Juice
Aloe Arborsecens

Recommended sites for you to explore:

http://www.cancertutor.com/
http://www.new-cancer-treatments.org/
http://phkillscancer.com/
http://curecancer73-don.blogspot.ca/2011/07/beating-cancer-by-don-porter.html
http://www.chrisbeatcancer.com/

http://www.budwig-videos.com/
http://drsircus.com/protocol-components
http://www.naturalnews.com/

Conclusion

I really want you to take a good long hard look around you, your loved ones and friends and see who has been stricken with cancer or some type of malady. Almost 1 in every 5th person will be stricken with some type of cancer. Does that not make you want to scratch your head and ask why? What has changed in the last several decades for this to happen?

I know personally before my father was diagnosed, I knew many and had heard of many with cancer and often the saying goes, "Omg, I am so sorry to hear this!" and then we go back to our normal routines.

It's up to you to start taking proactive action, take matters into your own hands. To put it frankly, "Nobody cares, other than you and your loved ones." You are the one that has to go home every day, endure the pain, the restless nights, the crying or being scared to death on whether or not you will live to see another day.

When the doctor states, "I have you in my best interest!" Bullshit! After that appointment he goes home to his family and does whatever he does. He is not the one that will be there with you to hold your hair while you're vomiting, or can't physically walk to the washroom, or have to deal with the physical and emotional stress that you're dealing with every single day while you still have a pulse. ***You're a 10 minute appointment at best!***

I wrote this book in the hopes that it would help at least a few people that do not know about other alternative therapies and that there is hope and you do have options. You do not have to rely on only your medical physician or oncologists for all the answers because they don't have all the answers.

You need to be your own advocate or have someone that is willing to act as one for you, when you are not capable. You can't be afraid to ask your doctor about supplements and natural cures. If he shows no interest, I personally would run in the other direction.

They have an obligation to answer your questions, any questions and in full detail until you fully understand the answer. This is YOUR LIFE! You don't have time to play around or be unsure or afraid of what he/she may think.

I urge you to do your research, really investigate the alternatives that are available to you because they are out there. Track down other cancer survivors and talk to them. They are out there!

One thing I wanted to explain and I am sure your all asking, "Well why didn't these protocol's or natural cures work for your father?"

My father was diagnosed with Stage 4 Small Cell Lung Carcinoma in October 2012 which is a very aggressive cancer that spreads fast. It had already metastasized to his lymph nodes in his throat. He was given 2 to 4 months to live with an option of 5 day radiation treatment to reduce the pain of the large tumor on his right lung.

He also had a small tumor on his right kidney, but upon diagnosis the initial tumor that was found on his right lung was already 8.5cm in diameter. It was rapidly growing into his rib cage which ultimately caused severe nerve damage and the majority of his pain.

After I had done some research into Vernon's protocol, baking soda/molasses, I fully explained everything to my father and he stated, "Let's do it!", "I am going to die anyway, what do we have to lose?"

After doing one round of the protocol my father started to feel better. Although during the break (we took about 2 weeks) he got extremely constipated and had not had a bowl movement for over 11 days. Most patients that are on heavy pain medication will experience constipation as one of the side effects.

Well this resulted in his first emergency room visit and 4 enemas later. He had lost so many fluids that night between the bowls and vomiting, it was incredible. I seriously did not think someone could hold that much within their body.

The emergency doctor then sent us home after being there for almost 8 hours even though my father's electrolytes were totally depleted and he could hardly walk.

This continued at home for another 2 days where my husband and I had to half carry him to the washroom due to the massive diarrhea, vomiting and weakness every few hours.

He was then taken back to the hospital where he stayed for 4 days to restore his electrolytes. Once back at home he was adamant that the baking soda protocol is what induced the constipation and refused to continue with anything. Due to the pain medications he was extremely confused most of the time. My father was very sensitive to the drugs as he had only ever taken Tylenol for his arthritis pain his entire life.

My father was on Dilaudid (Hydro morphine) and Fentanyl patches for the pain for over 2 months prior to this episode which ultimately was the culprit of the constipation.

The major play in all of this was that my father ended up with Hypercalcemia which only about 10-20% of lung cancer patients get. He just had to be the lucky one. It took us and the doctors exactly 6 to 7 weeks to figure this out due to his *extreme* behaviour change.

Hypercalcemia is when the cancer spreads to your bones which then starts attacking the bones, drilling holes in them which ultimately leeches out calcium into the blood stream. This also increases extreme bone and muscle pain. When your calcium levels reach between 3.5 to 4.0 the result is either coma or cardiac arrest.

Picture a boat (your bones) and the water (cancer) is constantly eating away at the structure. This is what hypercalcemia does. There are only 2 types of main medications that will plug the holes for a while, but eventually the medication wears off and ultimately the water sinks the boat. It is a very serious complication for cancer patients.

One major complication of Hypercalcemia is severe delirium and hallucinations. During the 8 months from diagnosis my father was lucid for about the first 4 months but with major confusion from the high pain medication he was on. From there it went downhill very quickly.

You have to be of sound mind to do these natural cures and protocols for them to work. 80% of the time my father thought he had a dead dog lying underneath the hospital bed we had setup in one of my living rooms, or that my statues teaky dolls (statues) were demons trying to kill him.

At times he even thought there was a time bomb strapped to his catheter tubing. He also experienced Sundowner's Syndrome which is awful. He would stay up for 4 or 5 days at a time and being incontinent at the same time and this continued for over 4 weeks.

So to be frank, there was no way I could be successful with any of these cures with my father as he was so stricken with these other complications. Every day it was a struggling battle, we never knew what would happened from one day to the next.

You have to be actively involved with your mind for these to work. I truly believe that if the hypercalcemia did not take hold of him, he would be sitting here with me today because he trusted me with every ounce of his body and mind, he made me his power of attorney for a reason. He knew I would fight for him and be his cheerleader. It came to a point where I had educated myself so much on his cancer and complications that I had to educate the EMS workers when they would arrive in regard to what Hypercalcemia was and the day and night time support workers as to his symptoms so they would understand if a problem had happened.

They would always ask me, "Are you a nurse?" I would just answer, "I am his daughter."

He had so much trust in me that when it came to his pills, food, water, appointments he would not listen to or trust anyone but me. When my mother or my husband would try to give him anything, his response would be, "Ask Kim first if it's ok."

My father wanted to live and we had made a pack together alone on that drive home from seeing his oncologist for the first diagnosis that we would fight this together and beat it. But sometimes things just don't work out the way we want them to.

If there is one thing you can do to better education yourself more on this matter than I urge you to watch these two films:

Food Matters
Hungry for Change

These film makers are just a few of the whistle blowers along with Mike Adams from NaturalNews.com and David Wolfe that is not afraid to expose to the public what is really going on with the Big Pharma, GMO'S and Cancer. I commend these people for informing the public and making them/us aware of what is truly going on today.

We need so many more people to join and fight this ongoing battle, but in the mean time we have to sit back and watch so many people die of cancer every single day even though there are cures.

I want to thank you for buying and reading my book. It means the world to me and would mean the world to my father, honestly!

If you could leave a review on Amazon where you purchased, I would be extremely grateful as this will help to get it into more hands that could use this information to either help themselves, a loved one or a friend.

I truly do hope that I have helped you in some small way or another.

P.S. I am in the process of writing my memoir of the 8 month ordeal that I went through with my father in great detail as his caregiver. There are many family or friend caregivers out there that are alone trying to care for someone with cancer and are at a breaking point. I know how hard it is and can relate first hand.

I want this memoir to help them know that they are not alone, that they are amazing, caring individuals that deserve to be recognized and that is why I am writing the book. I am hoping it will also close my chapter of morning, the pain, the anger and sadness that I still feel everyday.

If you are at all interested in the release date of any of my further books you can like my fanpage as I update it there everyday with new articles and information about my books that I will be releasing.

You can also message me there or any of the below links if you have any questions at all. I am more than happy to help in anyway that I possibly can.

https://www.facebook.com/LivingNaturallyRaw
http://livingnaturallyraw.com/
livingnaturallyraw@gmail.com

Much Love,
Kimberly